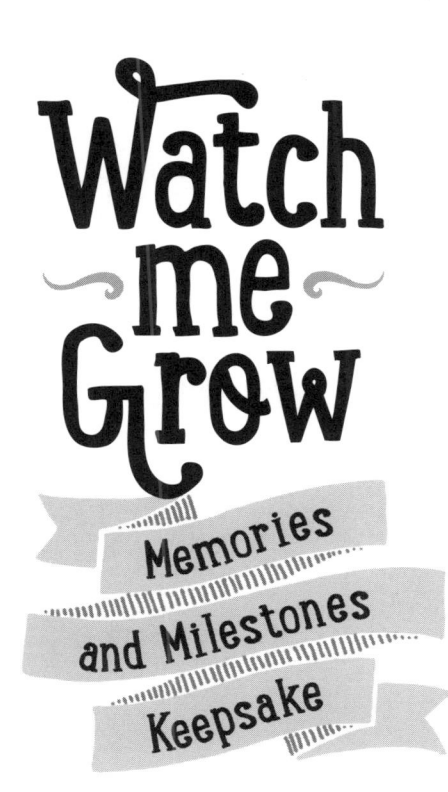

# Watch me Grow

## Memories and Milestones Keepsake

Created by
Michael Ball Jr.

Illustrated by
Pamela Goodman

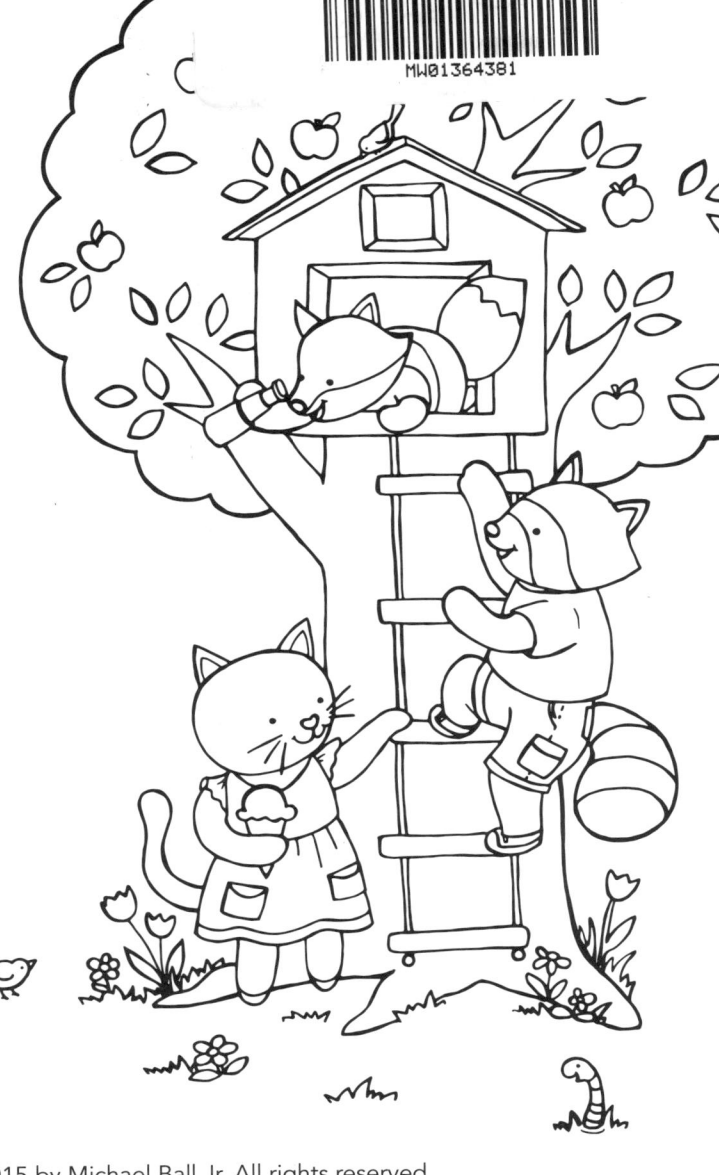

Edited by Karen A. Corekin, k.corekin@yahoo.com

Illustrations by Pamela Goodman, www.PamelaGoodman.com

Book design by Monica Thomas for TLC Graphics, www.TLCGraphics.com

.. Published by ..

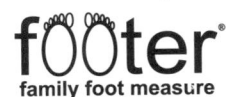

**footer**®
family foot measure

www.FootMeasure.com
Sister Bay, Wisconsin, USA

ISBN 978-0-692-34479-8
Printed in the United States of America

# How To Use This Book

**Watch Me Grow** is a wonderful way for families to track their child's growth and development together. Here is how to get started:

- Use tape or glue to attach a picture of your child on the next page. Be sure to include your child's name, birth date, and age.

- Complete your first measurement on the page marked *Year 1/Measurement 1*. Trace your child's foot in the blank area next to the height ladder with markers or crayons. You could even make a foot impression with paint for messy good fun! If you use paint, don't forget to allow time for it to dry.

- Measure your child's height, using the measuring tape included with your *Watch Me Grow* kit. Record the measurement on the height line. Your child can place the "I'm This Tall!" sticker to mark their height next to the ladder.

- Weigh your child on your home scale or at your child's next doctor appointment. Write the weight on the appropriate line.

- Use the Footer family foot measure® to get an accurate size for your child's foot. This is the perfect way to prepare for a trip to the shoe store or shopping online.

- Complete the measurement page. The adjacent page has fun questions for you and your child to answer; then your child can color the illustration.

- Repeat this process every 4 months and fill-in a new set of pages! Included are "It's f00ter time!" stickers that you can place on your calendar as a reminder.

Remind your child that this is a very special book and only one section at a time can be colored. If your child is really enjoying the process, have him or her draw and color other related pictures on plain paper to extend the activity.

## Examples of Milestones

Starting with *Year 1/Measurement 2*, you can fill in *Milestones Since My Last Measurement*. Maybe your child lost a tooth, began a new grade in school, or learned to ride a bike! Think of things you will want to remember about your child when you look back at this book.

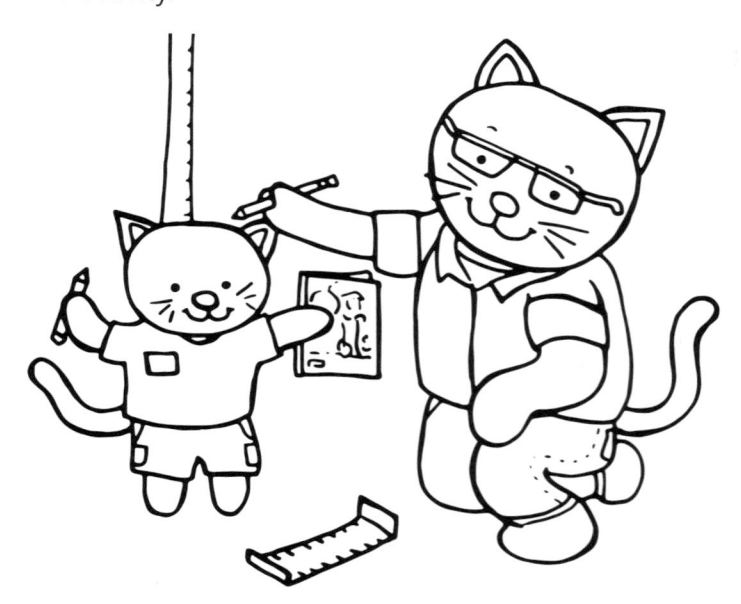

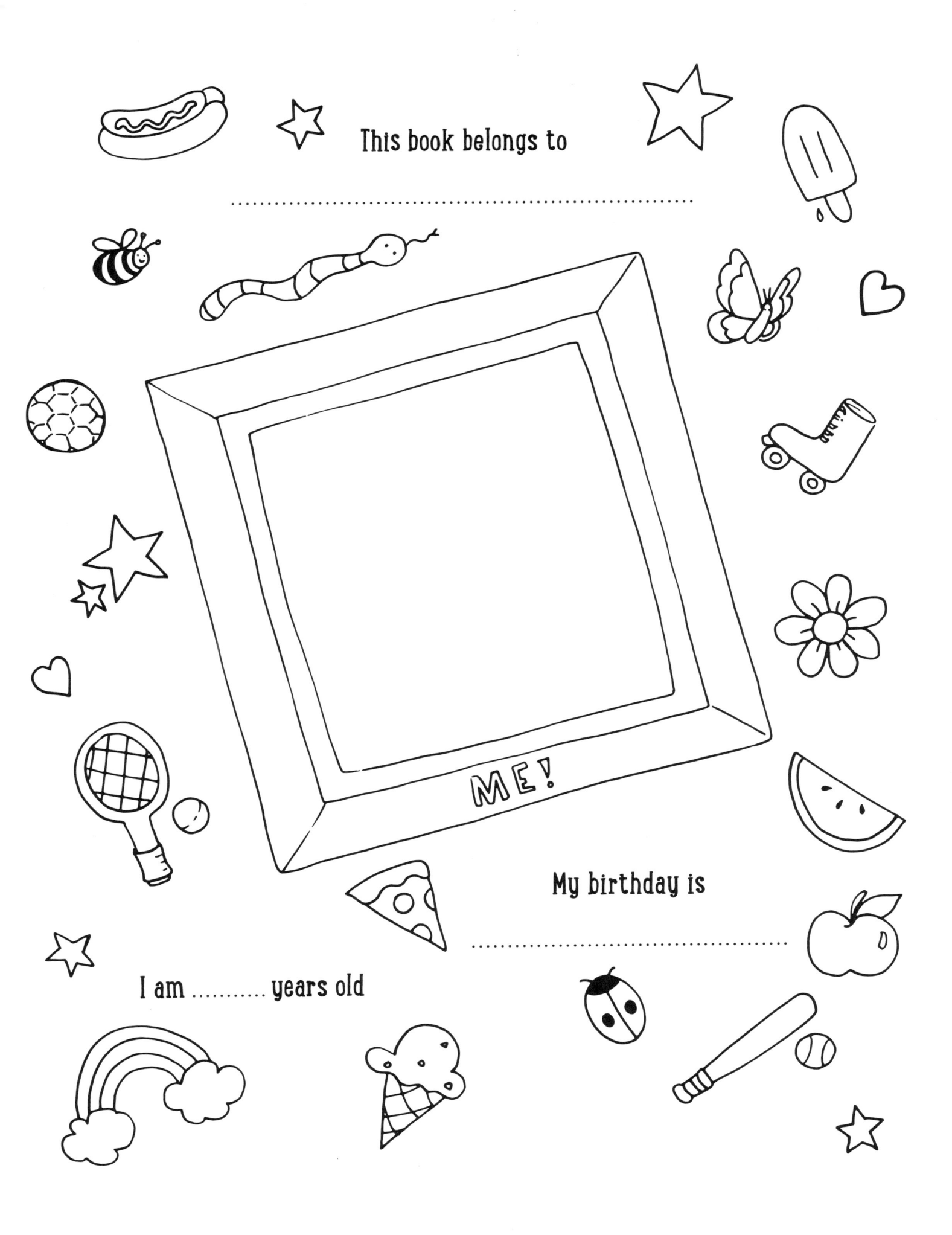

This book belongs to

..............................................

My birthday is

..............................................

I am ........... years old

ME!

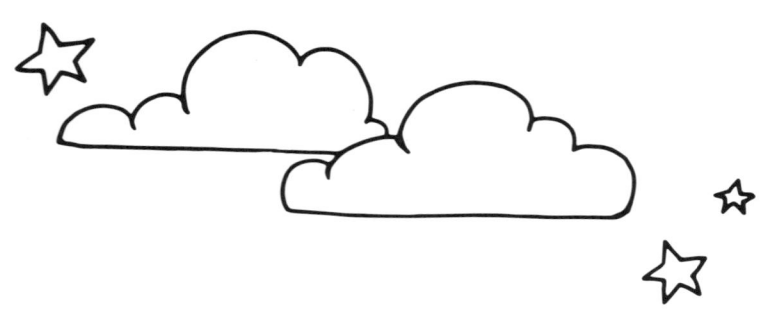

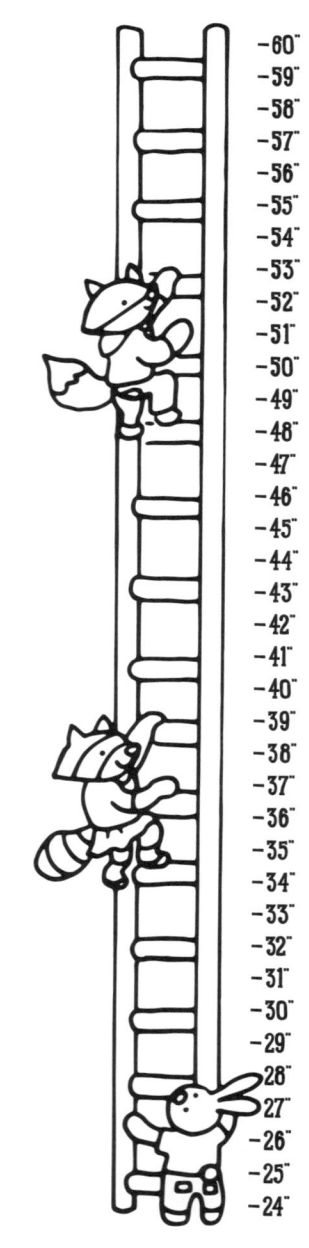

```
-60"
-59"
-58"
-57"
-56"
-55"
-54"
-53"
-52"
-51"
-50"
-49"
-48"
-47"
-46"
-45"
-44"
-43"
-42"
-41"
-40"
-39"
-38"
-37"
-36"
-35"
-34"
-33"
-32"
-31"
-30"
-29"
-28"
-27"
-26"
-25"
-24"
```

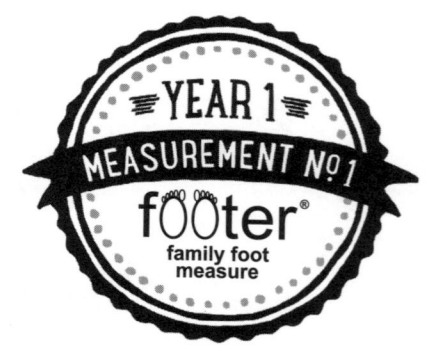

YEAR 1
MEASUREMENT №1
footer
family foot measure

Today is ............................. My height is ..............

My footer size is..............., and I weigh ...............

My favorite books are ..............................................

..............................................

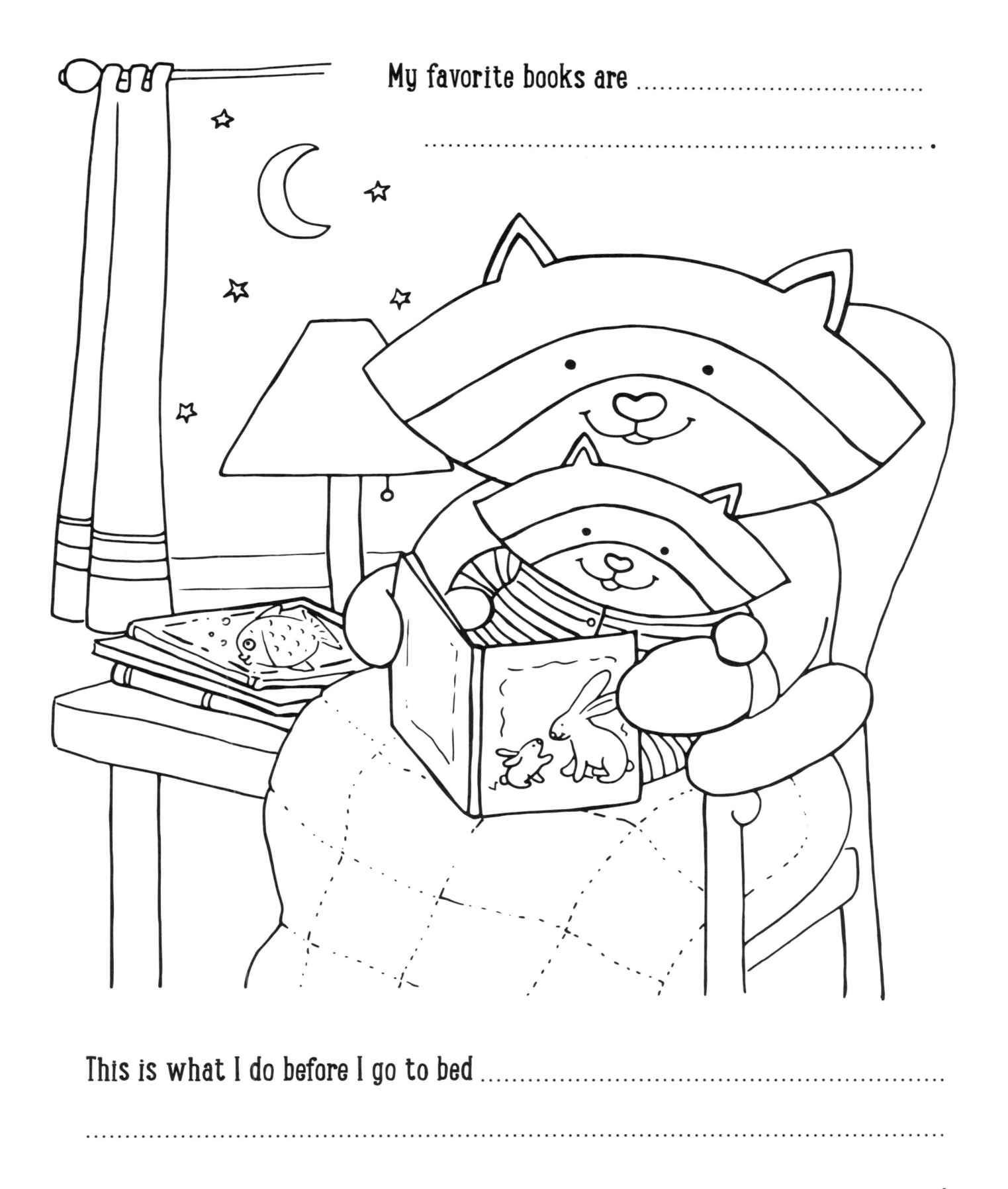

This is what I do before I go to bed ..............................................

..............................................

..............................................

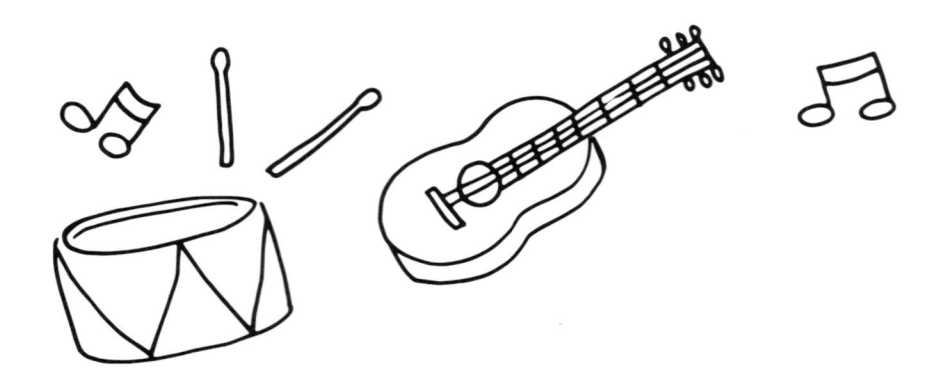

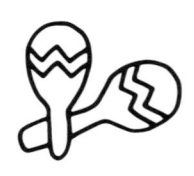

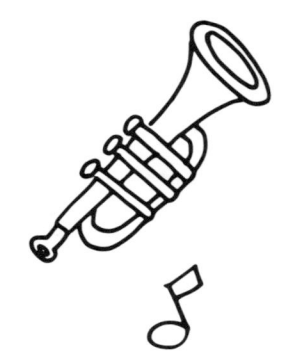

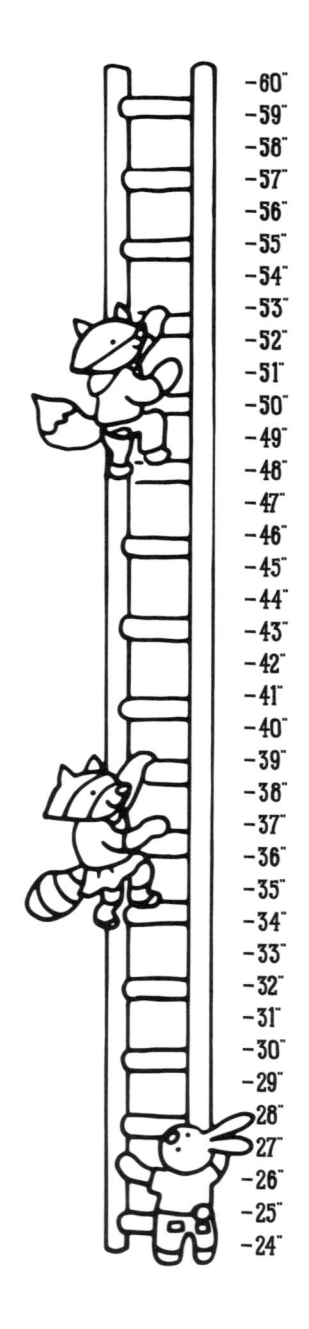

-60"
-59"
-58"
-57"
-56"
-55"
-54"
-53"
-52"
-51"
-50"
-49"
-48"
-47"
-46"
-45"
-44"
-43"
-42"
-41"
-40"
-39"
-38"
-37"
-36"
-35"
-34"
-33"
-32"
-31"
-30"
-29"
-28"
-27"
-26"
-25"
-24"

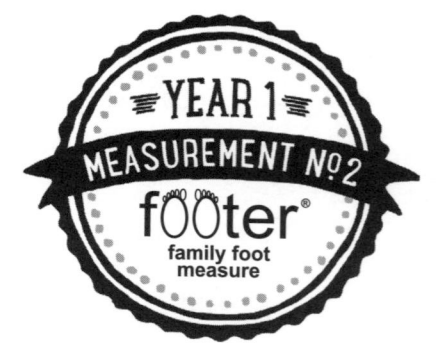

YEAR 1
MEASUREMENT Nº 2
foòter®
family foot
measure

Today is ........................... My height is .............

My foòter size is..............., and I weigh................

My favorite musical instrument is ................................................. .

My favorite songs are ...........................................................

...............................................................

Milestones since my last measurement

...............................................................

...............................................................

...............................................................

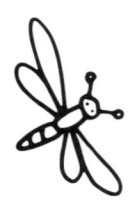
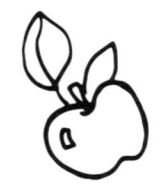
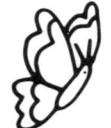
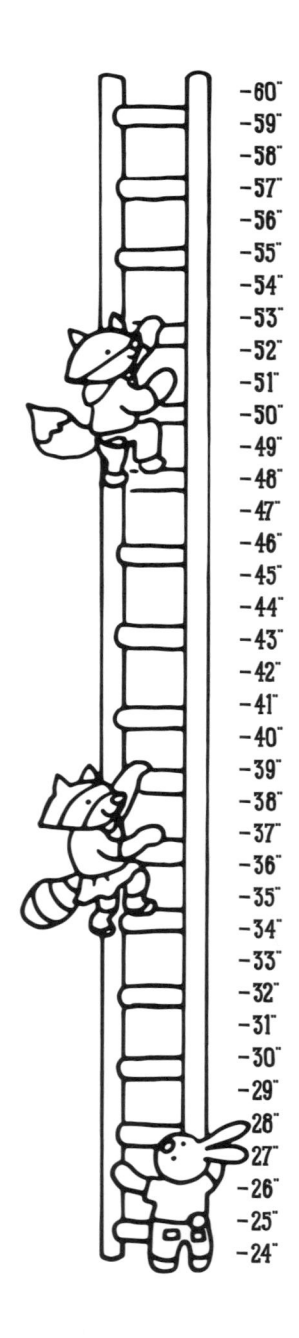

- 60"
- 59"
- 58"
- 57"
- 56"
- 55"
- 54"
- 53"
- 52"
- 51"
- 50"
- 49"
- 48"
- 47"
- 46"
- 45"
- 44"
- 43"
- 42"
- 41"
- 40"
- 39"
- 38"
- 37"
- 36"
- 35"
- 34"
- 33"
- 32"
- 31"
- 30"
- 29"
- 28"
- 27"
- 26"
- 25"
- 24"

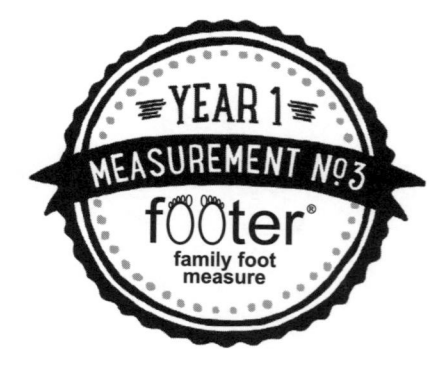

YEAR 1
MEASUREMENT № 3
footer®
family foot measure

Today is ............................. My height is ...............

My footer size is ..............., and I weigh ................

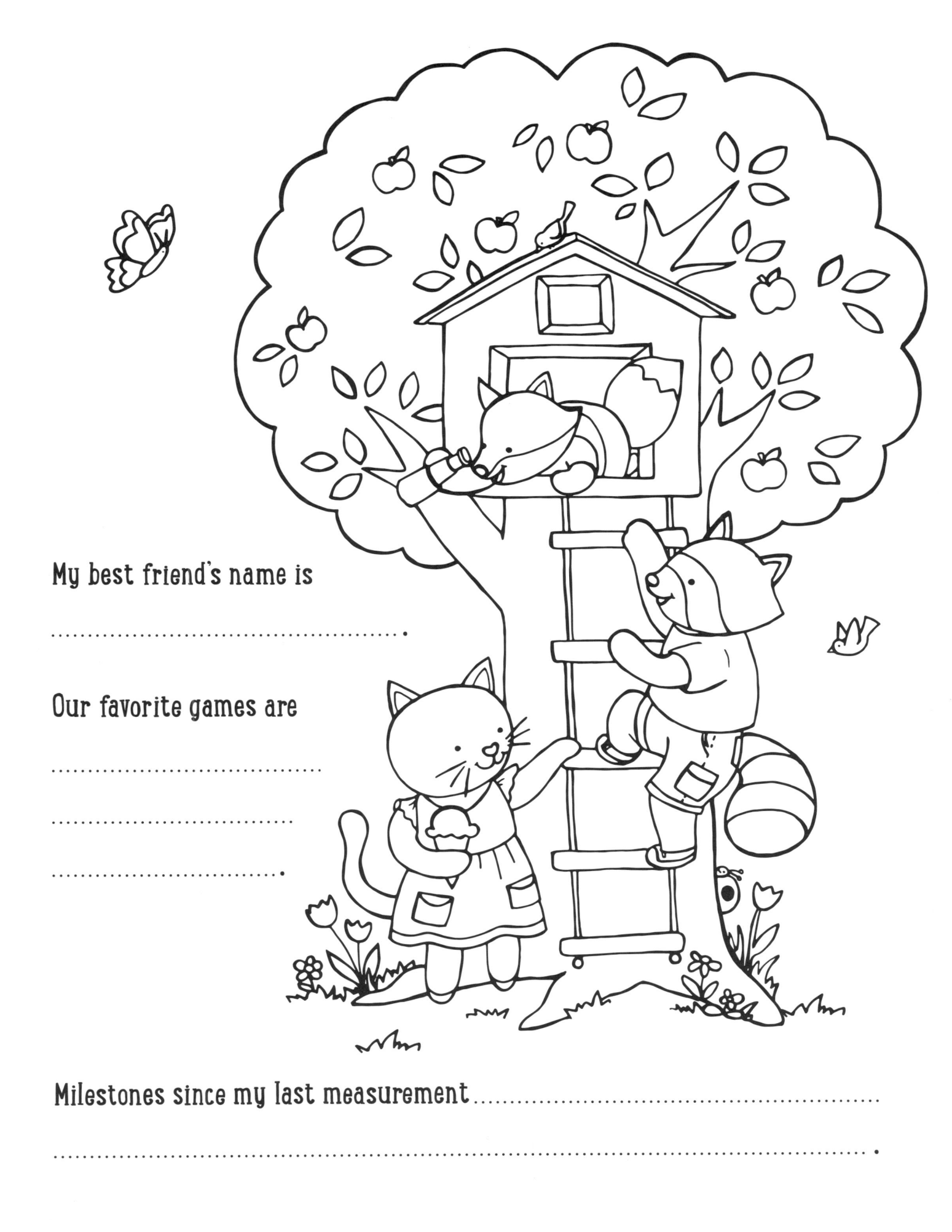

My best friend's name is

................................................

Our favorite games are

................................................

................................................

................................................

Milestones since my last measurement ................................................

................................................

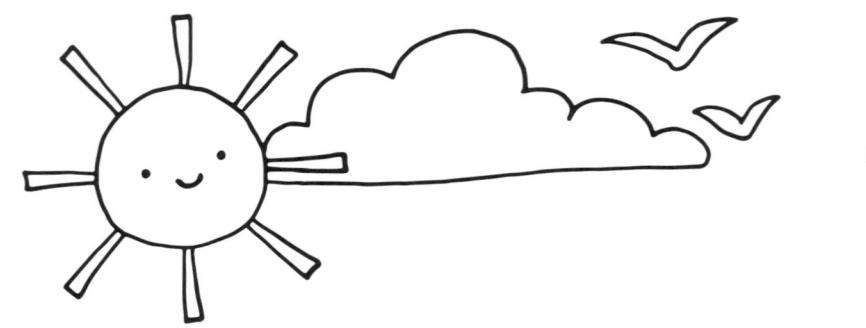
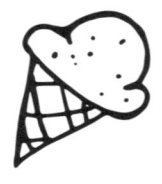

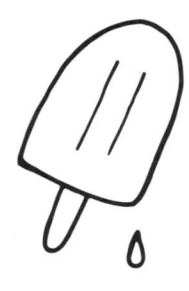
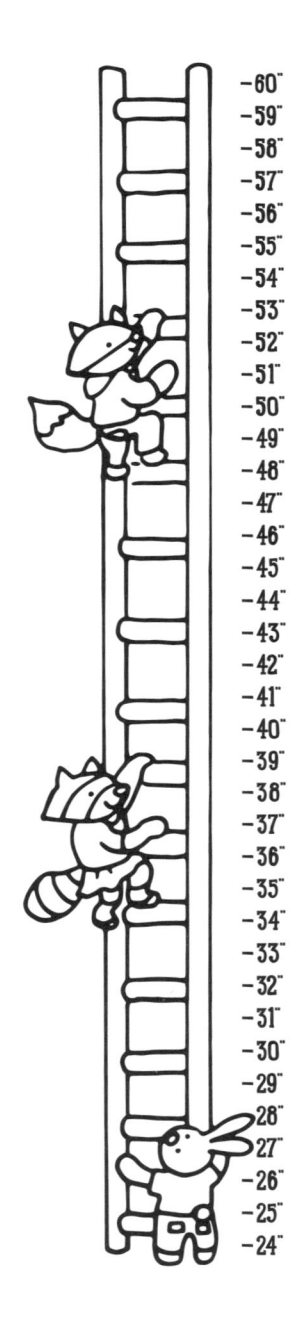

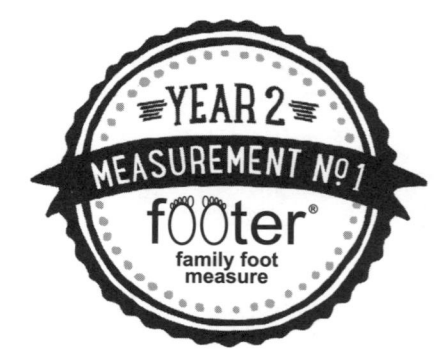

YEAR 2
MEASUREMENT Nº 1
fOOter®
family foot measure

Today is ........................ My height is .............

My fOOter size is.............., and I weigh...............

My favorite sweet treat is.............................................................. .

Meals I enjoy the most are

..........................................................................................

..........................................................................................

.................................................................................... .

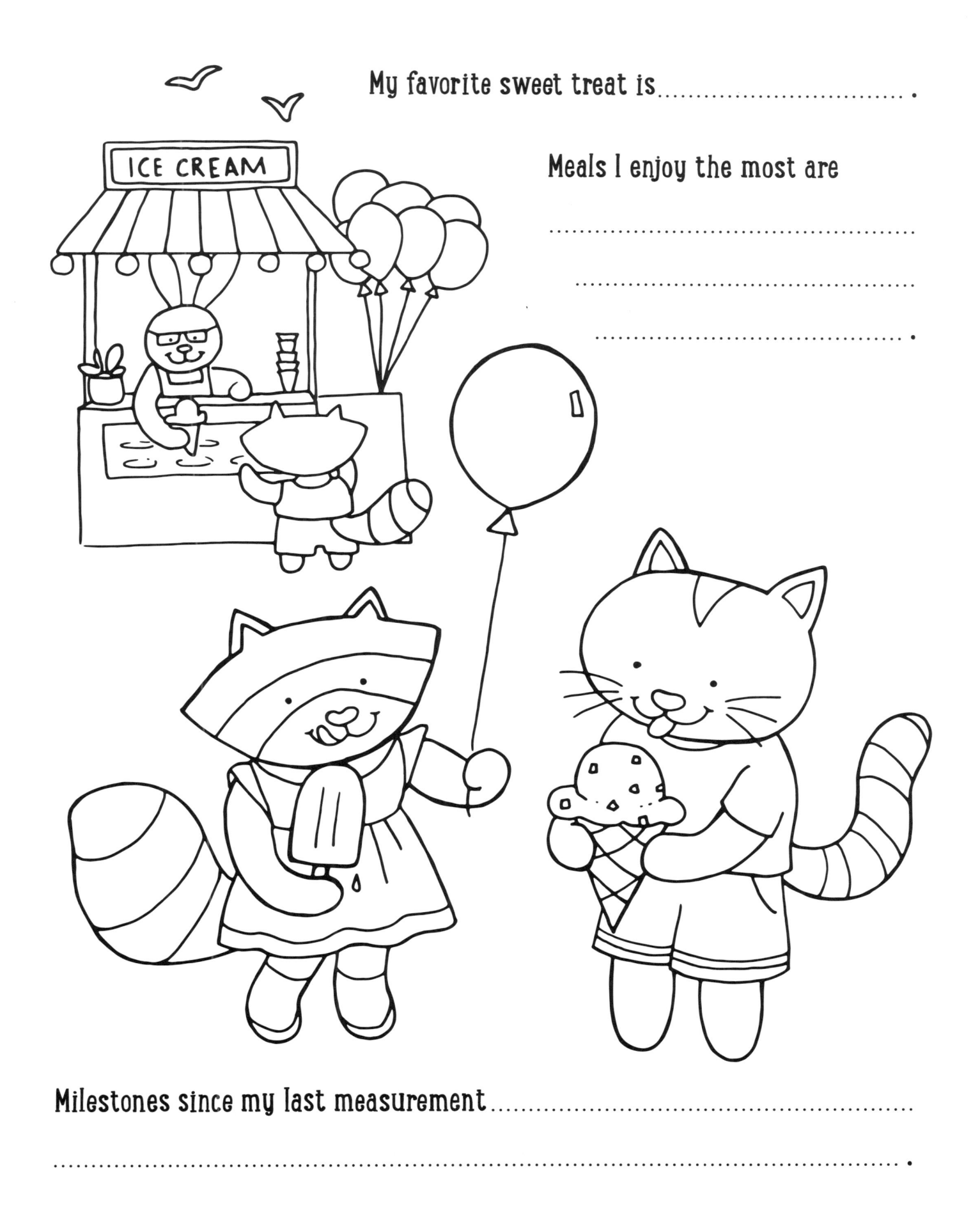

Milestones since my last measurement......................................................

.................................................................................................... .

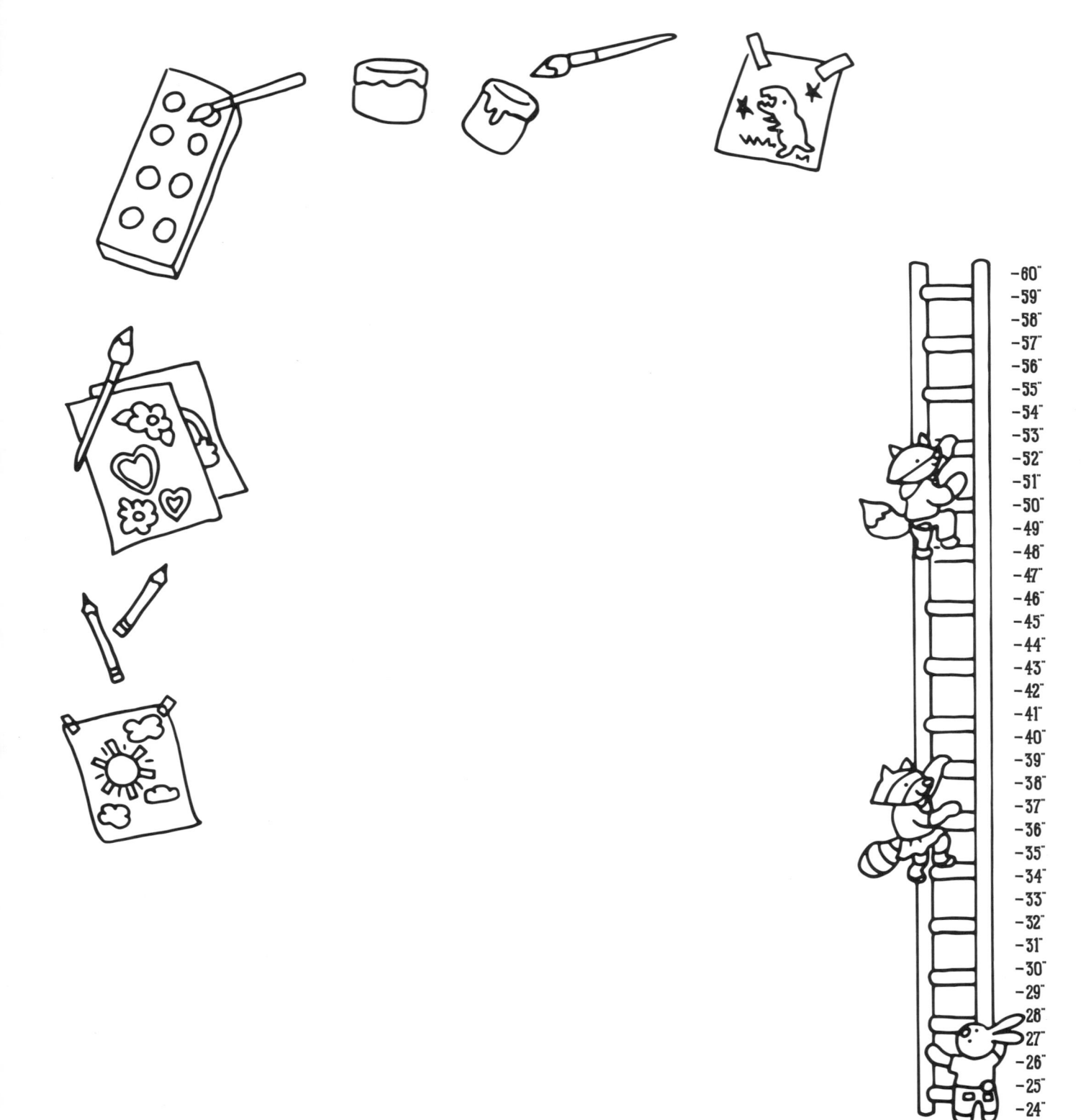

YEAR 2
MEASUREMENT Nº 2
fOOter®
family foot
measure

Today is ........................... My height is ..............

My fOOter size is................, and I weigh................

-60"
-59"
-58"
-57"
-56"
-55"
-54"
-53"
-52"
-51"
-50"
-49"
-48"
-47"
-46"
-45"
-44"
-43"
-42"
-41"
-40"
-39"
-38"
-37"
-36"
-35"
-34"
-33"
-32"
-31"
-30"
-29"
-28"
-27"
-26"
-25"
-24"

My favorite color is...........................................•

Things I like to draw most are.......................

.........................................................................

.........................................................•

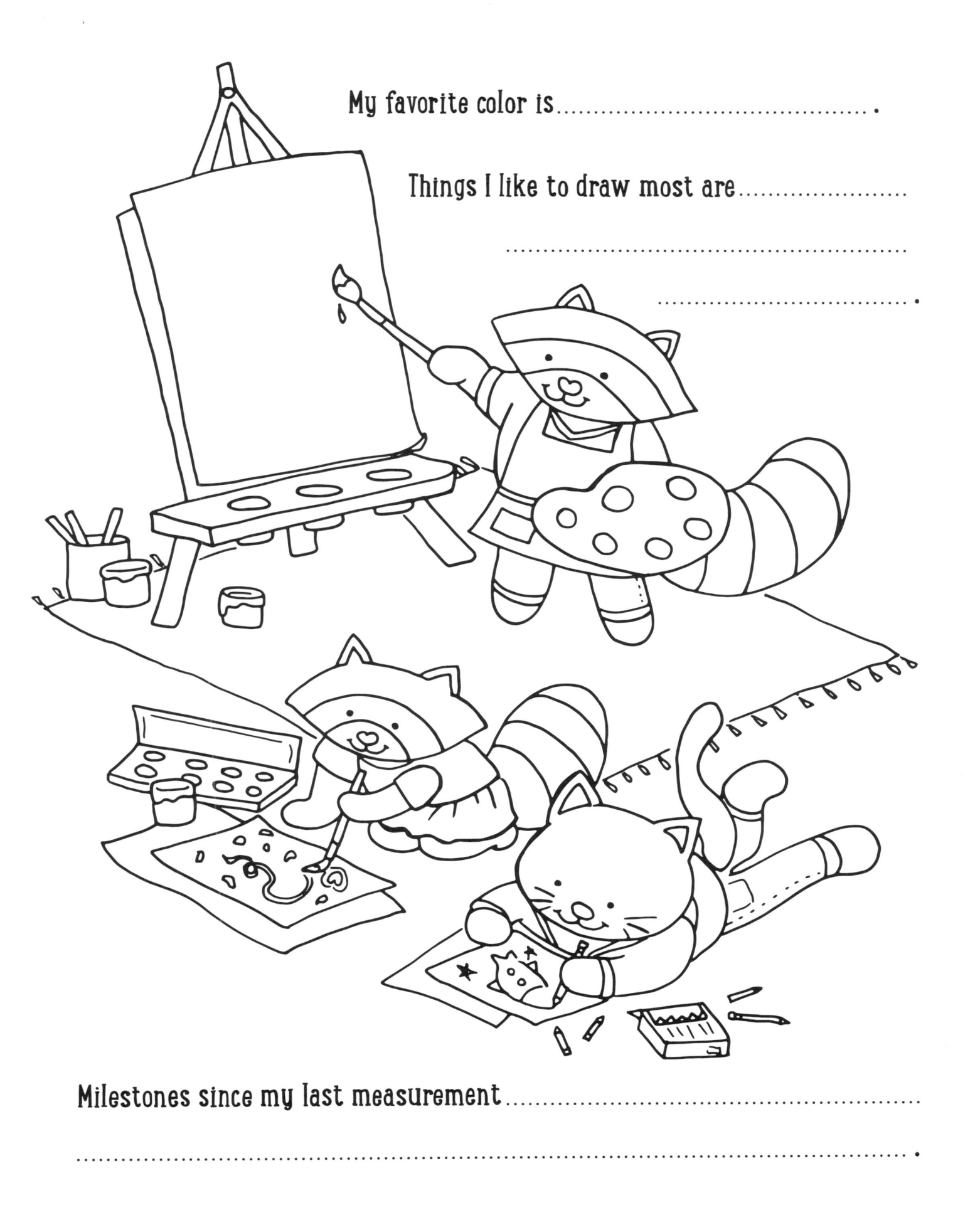

Milestones since my last measurement...........................................................

.........................................................................•

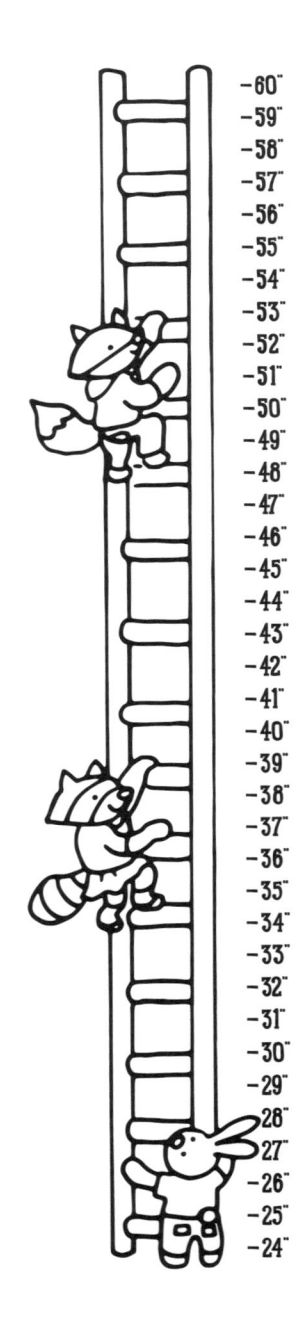

- 60"
- 59"
- 58"
- 57"
- 56"
- 55"
- 54"
- 53"
- 52"
- 51"
- 50"
- 49"
- 48"
- 47"
- 46"
- 45"
- 44"
- 43"
- 42"
- 41"
- 40"
- 39"
- 38"
- 37"
- 36"
- 35"
- 34"
- 33"
- 32"
- 31"
- 30"
- 29"
- 28"
- 27"
- 26"
- 25"
- 24"

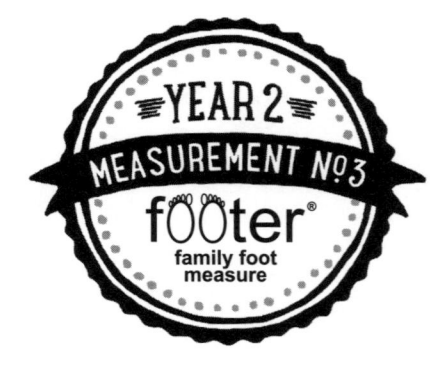

YEAR 2
MEASUREMENT Nº3
footer®
family foot
measure

Today is ........................... My height is ...............

My footer size is ..............., and I weigh ................

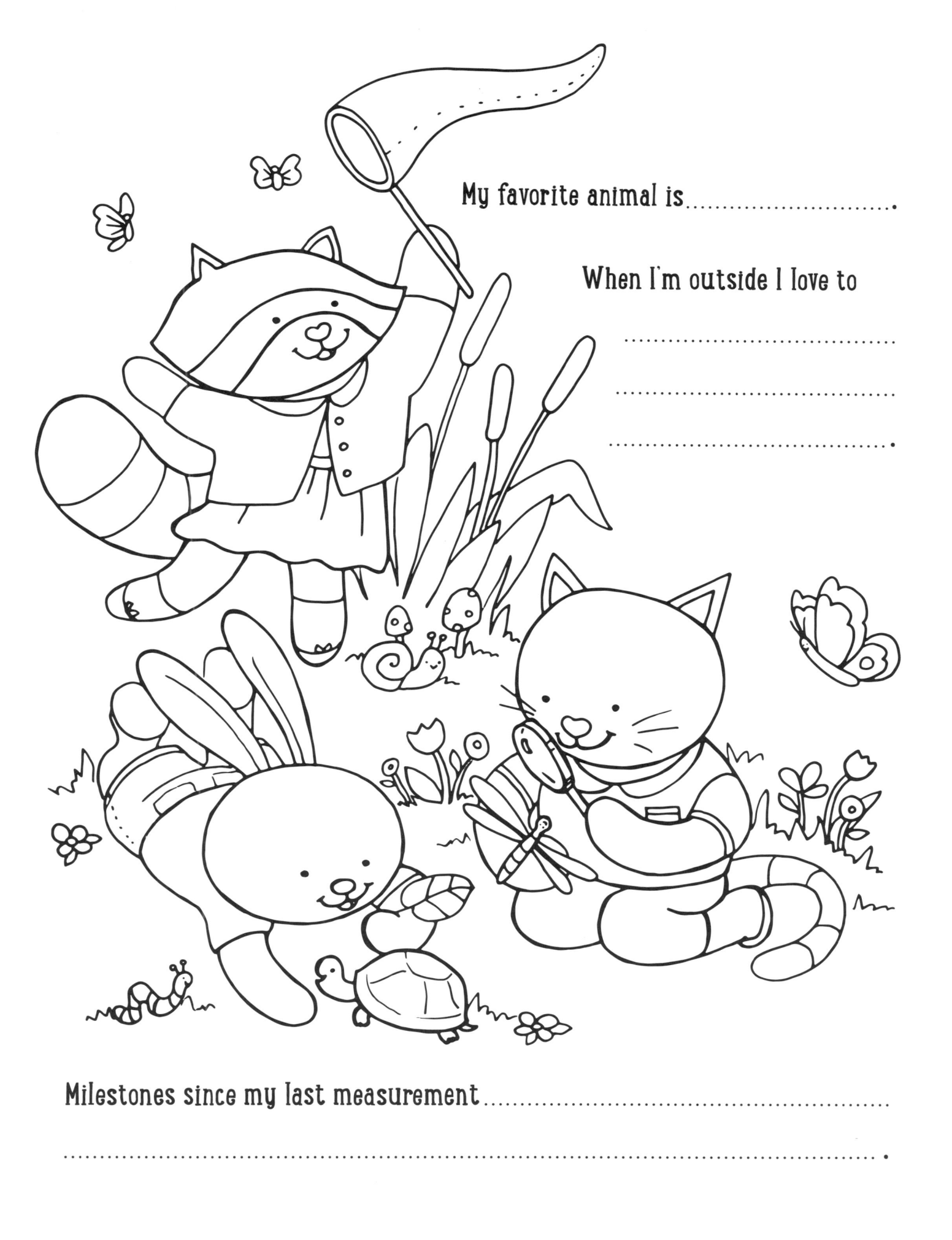

My favorite animal is ................................

When I'm outside I love to

...............................................

...............................................

...............................................

Milestones since my last measurement ...........................................................

...............................................................

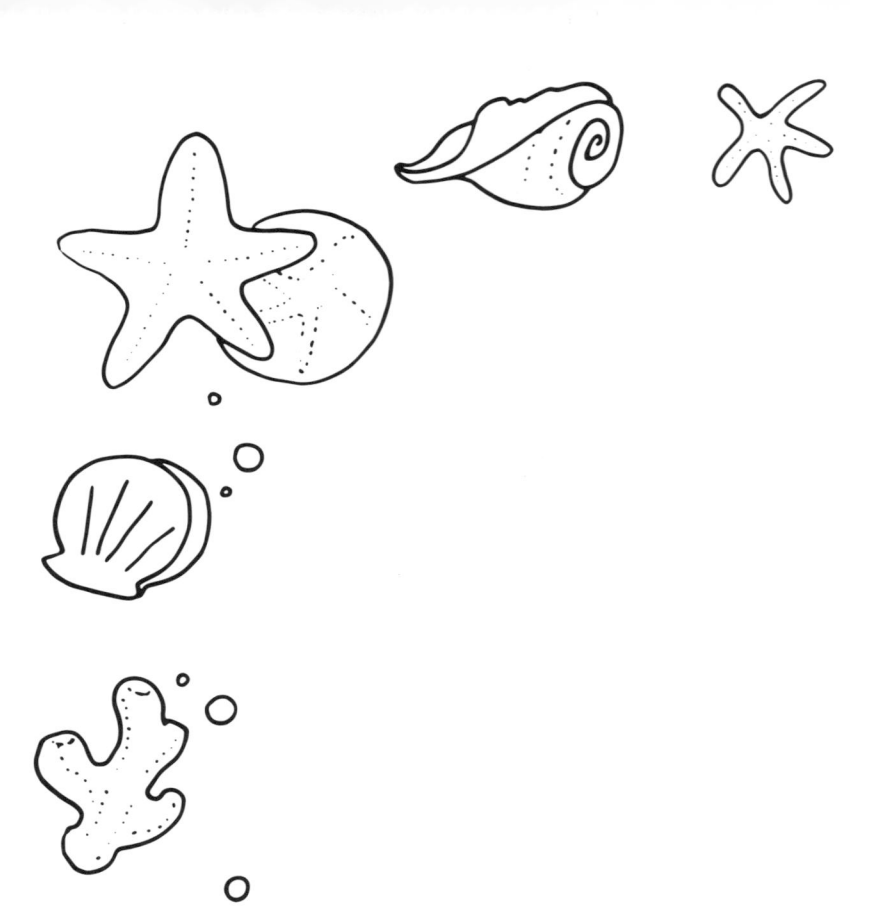

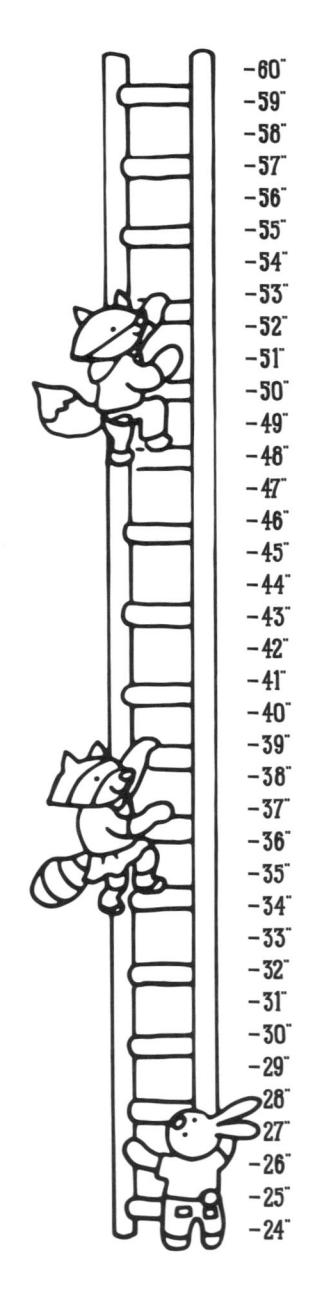

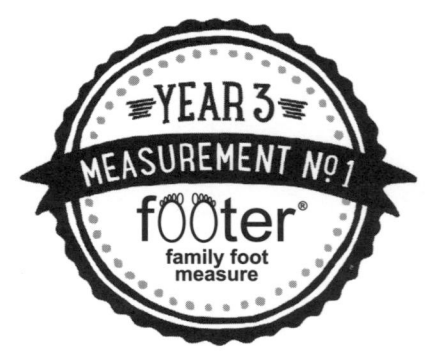

Today is ........................... My height is .............

My f👣ter size is ..............., and I weigh ...............

My favorite sport is .......................................

My favorite vacation spot is

....................................... .

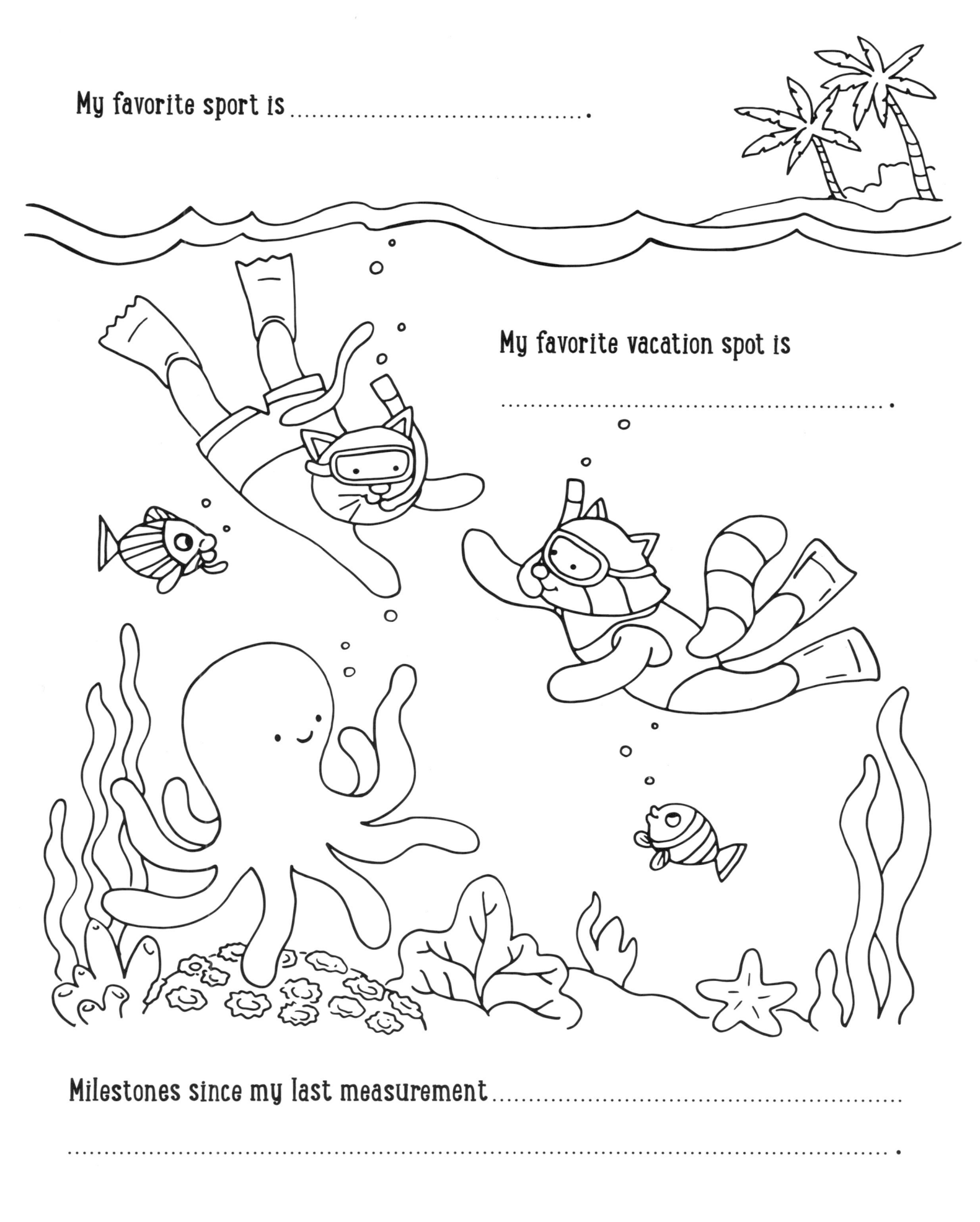

Milestones since my last measurement .......................................

....................................... .

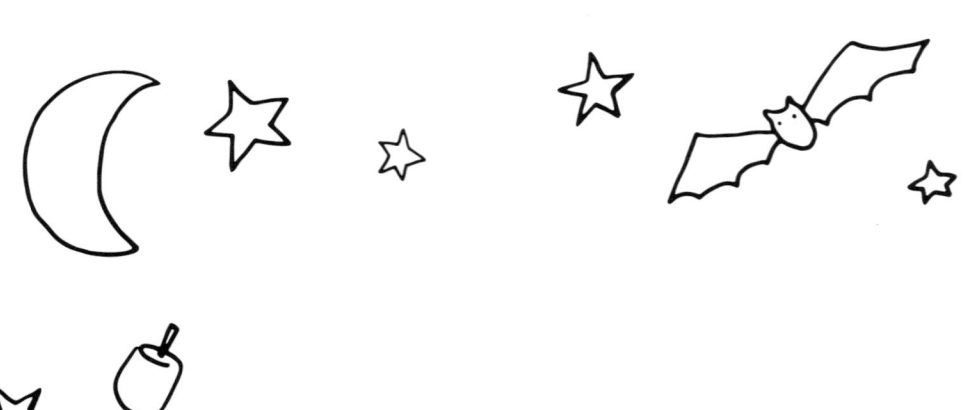

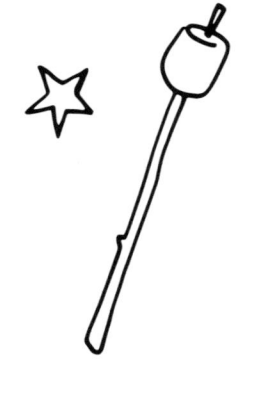

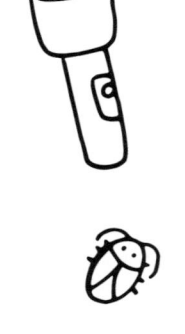

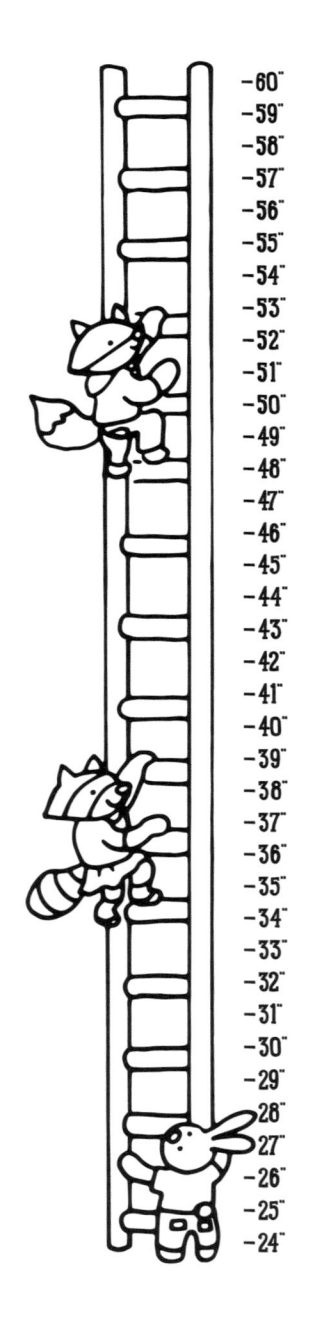

-60"
-59"
-58"
-57"
-56"
-55"
-54"
-53"
-52"
-51"
-50"
-49"
-48"
-47"
-46"
-45"
-44"
-43"
-42"
-41"
-40"
-39"
-38"
-37"
-36"
-35"
-34"
-33"
-32"
-31"
-30"
-29"
-28"
-27"
-26"
-25"
-24"

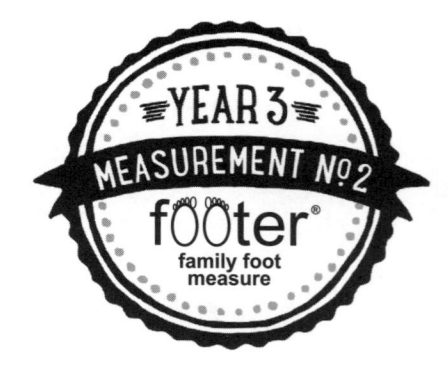

**YEAR 3**
**MEASUREMENT № 2**
footer®
family foot measure

Today is ........................... My height is ..............

My footer size is..............., and I weigh...............

My favorite camping activities are

..................................................................

..................................................................

.................................................... .

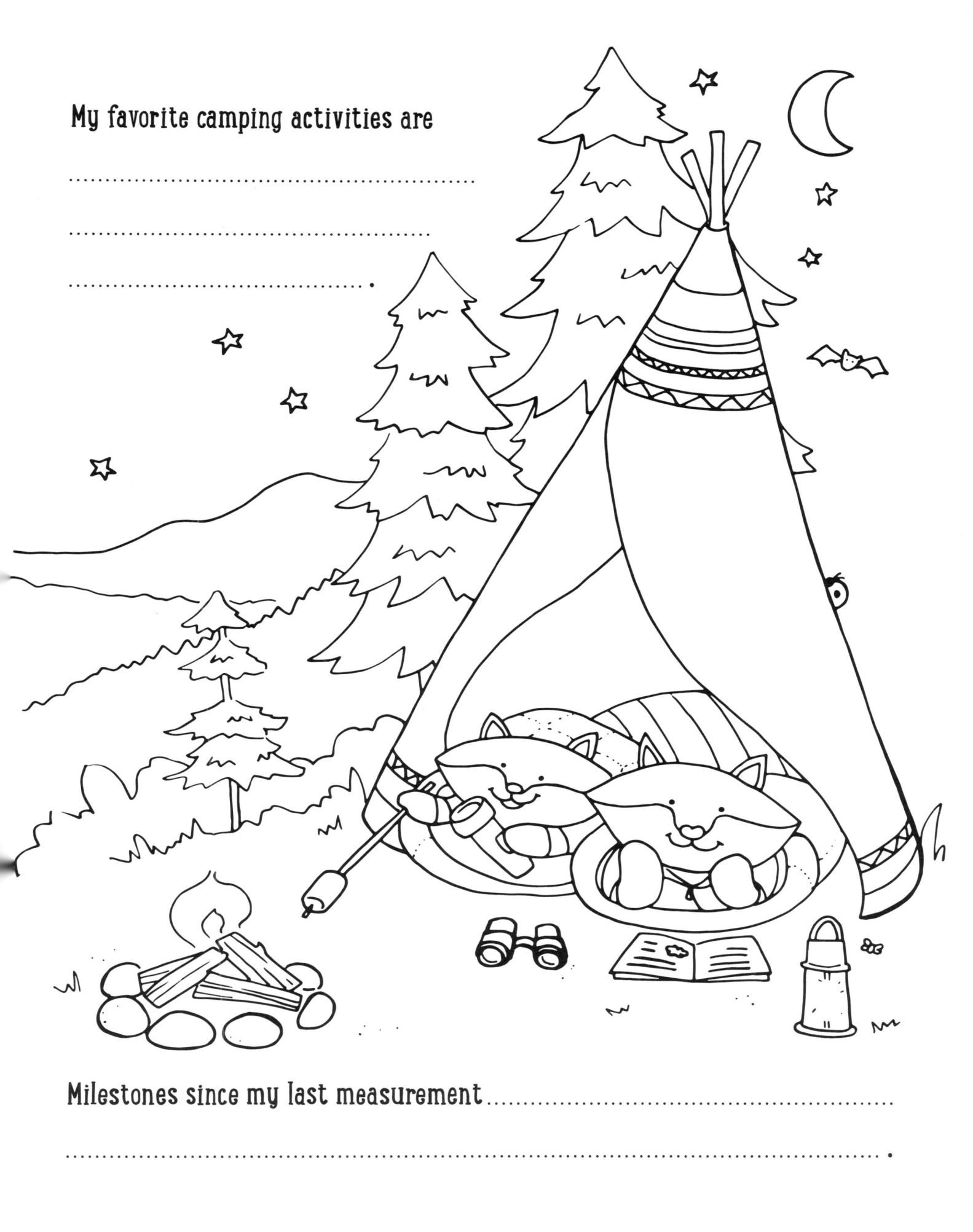

Milestones since my last measurement ...............................................................

.................................................................. .

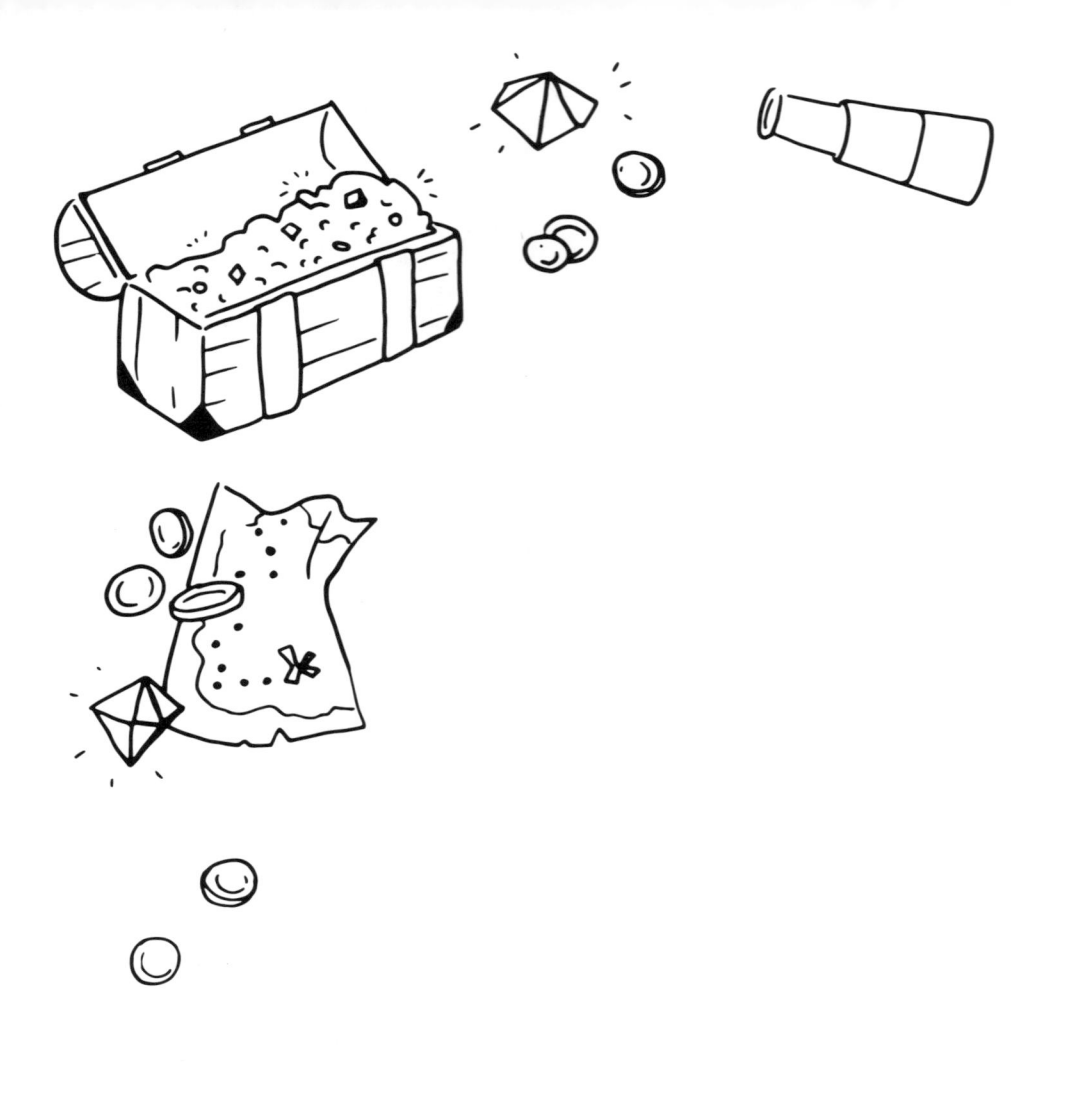

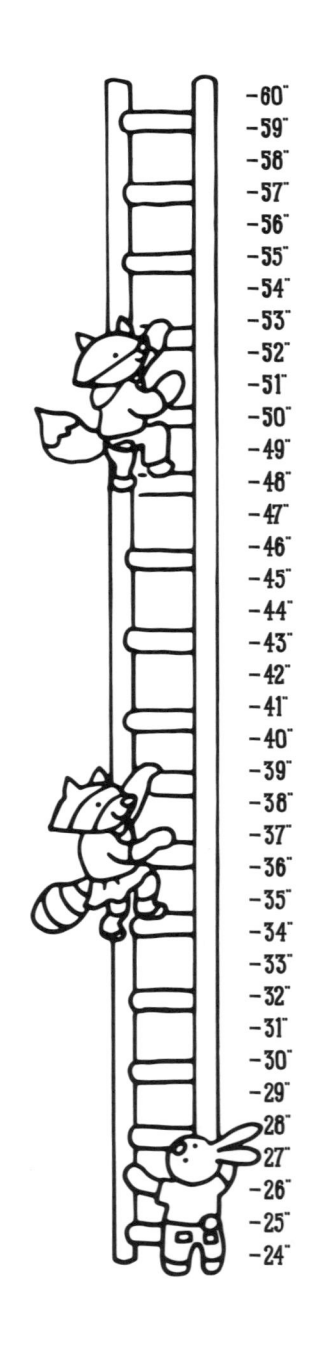

Height scale (inches): -60", -59", -58", -57", -56", -55", -54", -53", -52", -51", -50", -49", -48", -47", -46", -45", -44", -43", -42", -41", -40", -39", -38", -37", -36", -35", -34", -33", -32", -31", -30", -29", -28", -27", -26", -25", -24"

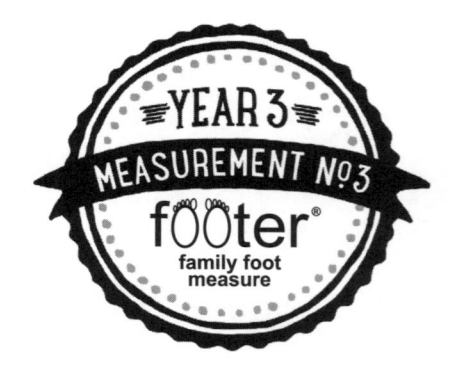

YEAR 3
MEASUREMENT Nº3
fOOter®
family foot measure

Today is ........................... My height is .............

My fOOter size is..............., and I weigh ...............

My favorite movie is ........................................................................ .

When I grow up I want to be

......................................................................................................

......................................................................................................

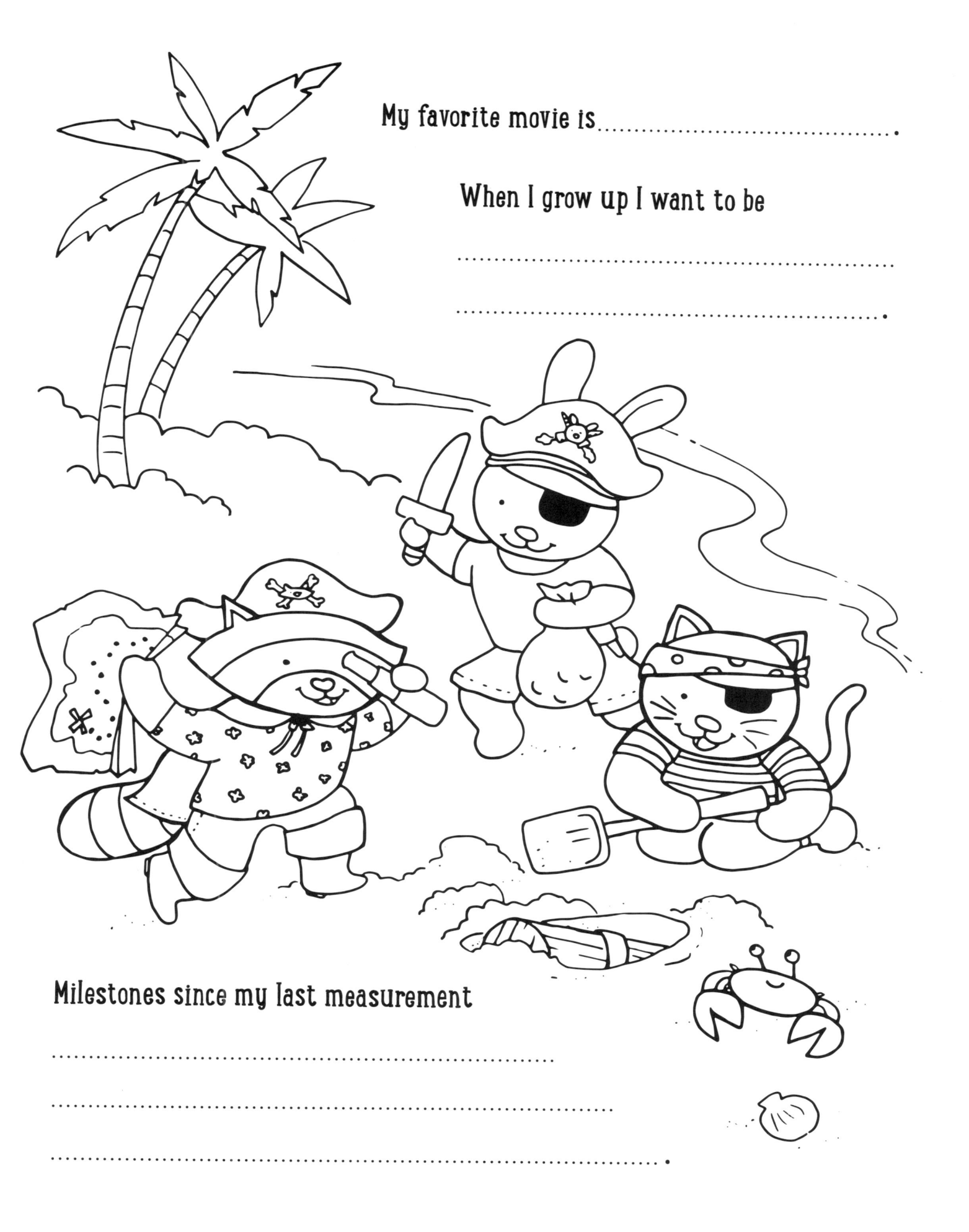

Milestones since my last measurement

......................................................................................................

......................................................................................................

......................................................................................................

# Look How I've Grown

## Memories and Milestones

The date of my first measurement was

........................................................................

and my last was...............................

I grew..........inches and my footer

size went from..........to..........!

........................................................

........................................................

........................................................

........................................................

........................................................

........................................................

........................................................

........................................................

........................................................

........................................................

........................................................

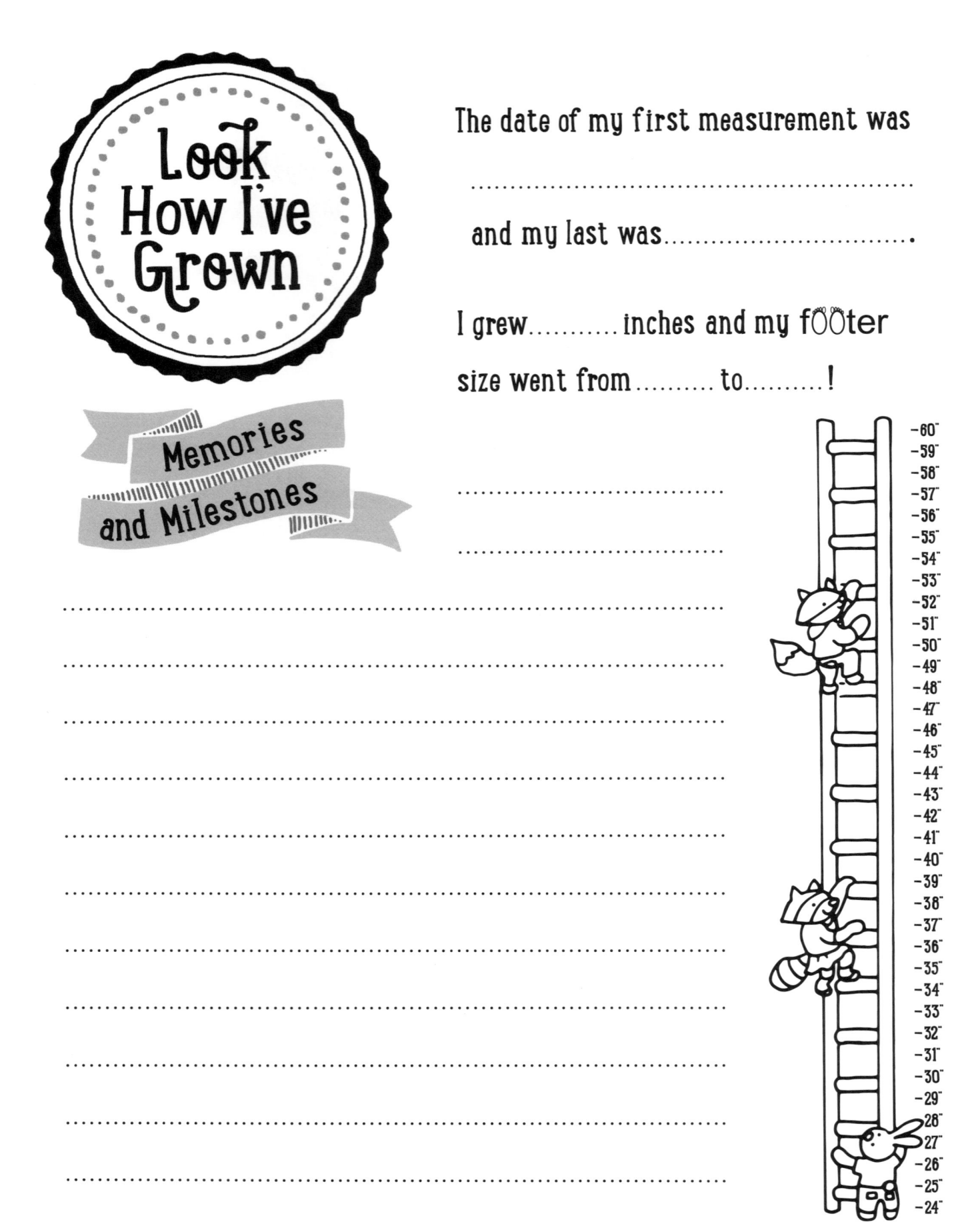

ME!

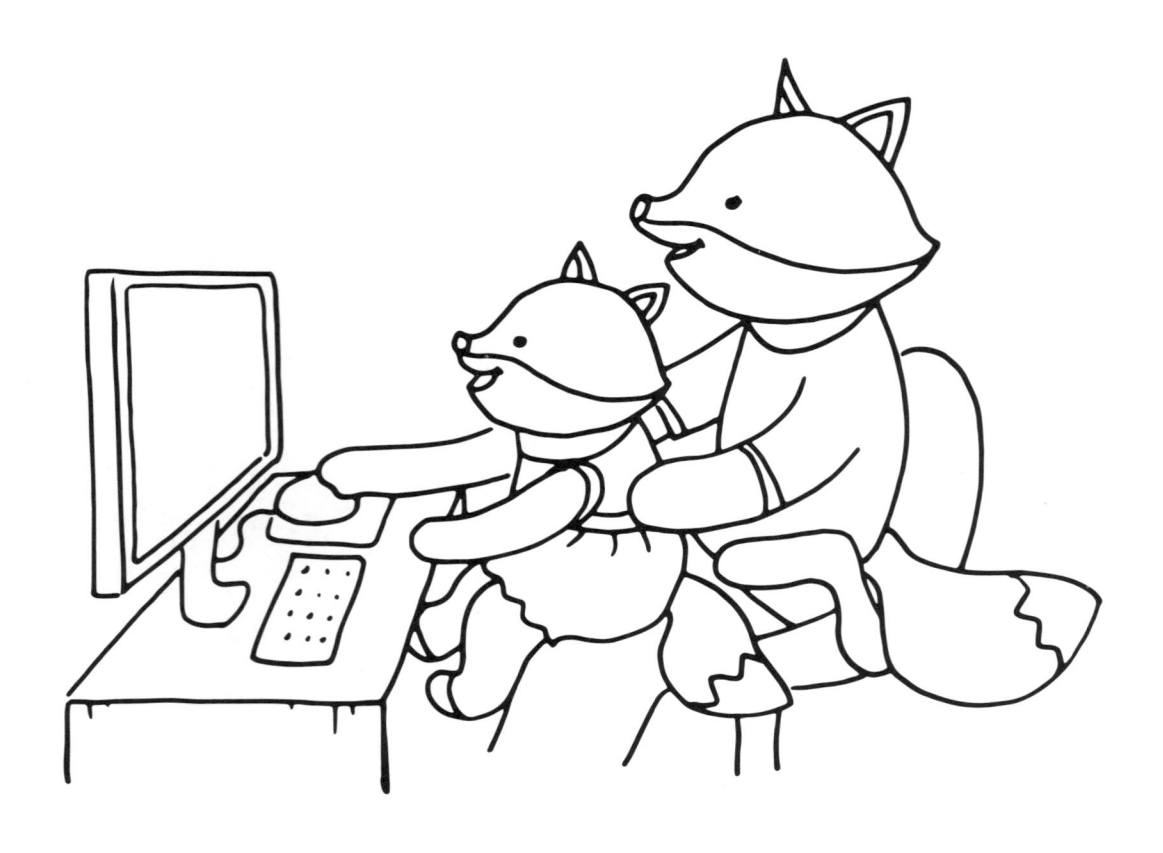

If you would like additional copies of *Watch Me Grow*
or to buy a Footer family foot measure®, visit us at
**www.WatchMeGrowBook.com** or **www.FootMeasure.com**.